Be Transformed...

...By the Renewing of Your Mind

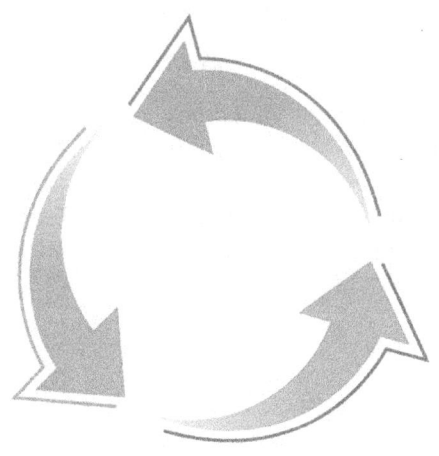

Ana Kerner

BE TRANSFORMED...
BY THE RENEWING OF YOUR MIND

ISBN-10: 1530855926
ISBN-13: 978-1530855926

Cover design by Ana Kerner

The following were referred to for Bible quotations:

The Holy Bible in Hebrew and English, Copyright 2014 The Bible Society in Israel

The Scriptures, Copyright 2012 by the Institute for Scripture Research, South Africa

Langenscheidt Pocket Hebrew Dictionary to the Old Testament, Hebrew English, by Dr. Karl Feyerabend, Printed in Germany

Student's Hebrew and Chaldee Dictionary to the Old Testament, compiled by Alexander Harkavy, Hebrew Publishing Company, New York, 1914

Buy My Books At: www.amazon.com

Contact Me At: annsart29@gmail.com

Self published through Createspace.com

DEDICATION

I dedicate this book

to all who have suffered mentally,

whatever the condition and whatever the cause.

And to our All-Knowing,

Loving God

Who allows our suffering.

May you receive your healing from

our Almighty Creator,

as I have.

CONTENTS

LAYING THE FOUNDATION

"I urge you...
by the mercies of God,
to present yourselves
as a living sacrifice,
set apart and pleasing to God,
as your service to Him
which is
from the heart."

Romans 12:1

The keys to the healing I have experienced are simple.

But they require certain qualities such as humility and complete submission to God and His Word. These things are not easy for anyone to come by. You cannot submit to God unless you trust him with all your heart and being.

What I am about to tell you will certainly be a challenge but it is not beyond anyone's reach. You have to want it. You have to learn to be disciplined.

You will need to learn to pray and you will need to have your own Bible in order to put, what I am about to tell you, into practice.

What I write in this book will be a benefit to ANYONE, not just someone with a head injury. But I will focus on those who have suffered a Traumatic Brain Injury because this is what I have been healed from and perhaps by telling my story, others will get their healing too.

I have been to some doctors over the years, but the majority of my healing has been by the revelation of God as I have trusted in Him. I will explain this further later on. This has actually been a blessing because I have learned many things from God Himself and several doctors have since benefited from what I have learned.

One of my doctors, after hearing my story said, "You learned so much by what you have gone through that I think everyone should have a head injury once in their life!"

Another one of my doctors asked me to write this book so he could use it with his patients.

I can only thank our Almighty Creator God for healing me. Some of my healing came in an instant but most of it came through a lot of struggle over time. Both are from Him and Him alone.

Now I will start my story...

After reading the whole Bible at age twelve, I came to the decision to trust God's Word completely. I realized, even at that age, that the church I was attending did not teach everything as I read it in the Bible.

Was I to trust the church (man) or the Bible (God)?

I chose God and in the Bible, His Word.

At the same time I remember praying three life changing prayers.

1. I said, "God, if Your Word is true I want You to prove it true in my life."

2. I had read how the sins of the parents are passed on to the third and fourth generation so I prayed, "God, no matter what it takes, I ask that you break all the sins of my forefathers in

ME."

3. I realized we all have only one life to live so I asked, "God, I want my life to count. I don't want to waste it. Please use me for Your glory. I don't care what I have to go through. I just want my life to count for all eternity and for it to bring You glory. Oh, yes, and PLEASE do not let my life be boring!"

These are not prayers every twelve year old prays. These are not prayers many adults ever pray. But these prayers will make all the difference in a person's life, if you have the courage to pray them. I say courage because what happens after you pray such prayers will not be easy for anyone.

By praying like I did, you will be offering yourself as a living sacrifice to Almighty God. This means your life is no longer your own...

MY STORY BEGINS

"For we are His workmanship,
created in Messiah Y'shuah (Jesus)
for good works,
which God prepared beforehand
so that we would walk in them. "

Ephesians 2:10

God has done a lot of miracles in my life. Many are miracles of healing. What I am about to tell you in this book can bring miracles into your life too.

Like I mentioned, I was asked to write this book at the request of one of my doctors. He told me that of all the patients he has ever seen, none has exhibited such drastic healing as I have. Not just physical healing but mental, emotional and spiritual healing as well.

There is a good reason for this, I believe. I have to go into a little of my background in order for you to understand this book and in order for you to experience healing as I have.

As a very young child, I had a relationship with God and His Messiah, Y'shuah (Jesus). My parents taught me many prayers even before I was three years old so, truly, I have no memory apart from God being in my life.

After first reading the Bible at age twelve, I kept on reading it. God has been my constant companion since I was taught to pray as a toddler. I was always "talking" to Him inside of me. I know He was always with me.

When I was fourteen years old, I was thrown off of a horse,

riding bareback. I didn't know this horse had been used in rodeos and I wasn't prepared for her to buck suddenly like she did. Her mane had also been shaved so when she bucked I had nothing at all to hold on to.

I was thrown violently to the ground, landing on my forehead. I ended up needing a hundred stitches to repair the outer physical damage. But what had happened inside my head was not so easy to "patch up".

Before this accident, school had been easy. Not only was I a grade ahead for my age but the work was not even too challenging. I had been in the "high" math classes since the seventh grade, one of only three girls in the class of close to twenty five students.

All this changed in a moment's time.

Now, let me ask you something. If I had committed my life to God as a young child, why did I suffer a severe head injury? Was that God's will? Was the Adversary trying to "take me out" so I couldn't be used by God?

All I know is that God allowed it.

I knew the prayers I had prayed when I was twelve, so no matter what else was going on, I knew God had allowed it. I did not doubt this because He was my constant companion and friend. Therefore I never asked God, "Why?" or "Why me?"

In fact, I remember laying in my bed, my blackened eyes swollen shut, thanking God that he was allowing ME to go through this and not one of my brothers or sisters. I wouldn't want them to experience what I was going through. I didn't WANT to go through this either! It was not easy, to say the very least. But I had faith and I knew the prayers I had prayed.

So I continually asked God, "What are You trying to teach me now? What can I learn from this?"

If you want to get what God has for you in life, in every situation, you have to ask the right questions. Not, "Why me?" But, "What are You trying to teach me through this?" This will make all the difference in the outcome of your times of struggle.

What could God be teaching me through a head injury? What could He be teaching you?

First off, humility. Being smart, being intelligent, has it's downside and that is pride. When you are able to think in ways most others don't you can easily set yourself above them. This is not of God. Sometimes He needs to "knock us down" for our own good!

Then there is trust. Learning to trust God when you don't know "why" is an important lesson to learn. A lesson that will serve you well the rest of your life!

Also, perseverance. The ability to persevere is not something everyone can do in a difficult situation, especially keeping a good attitude while you do it.

And there is compassion. When YOU suffer with the right mindset, you will learn to have more compassion for others who are suffering too.

The Bible also says, in 1 Peter 4:1, "he who suffers in the body ceases from sin." Let me tell you, when you are suffering you have no desire to sin! You just want to make it through the day! Understanding this is quite amazing, actually, because it means that when God allows someone to suffer He can actually be PROTECTING them from sin or evil. A blessing in disguise!

We also become more tolerant of things. Tolerant of disruptions, tolerant of other people's differences, tolerant of changes in plans, and the list goes on. By learning to be more tolerant you learn to be more content. We are to be content in whatever situation we find ourselves in.

11

One of the biggest lessons a person can learn from suffering, to become a grateful person! How many people have no sense of gratitude? Most people tend to take a lot of things for granted. But when you go through a time of suffering you become thankful for even the "smallest" things. I say "smallest" but that is really a misnomer. In truth nothing is "small". Our lives are in a perfect balance and if anything at all is out of order it can affect a person in very big ways. Take sleep for instance. How many people thank God for the blessing of the ability to fall asleep? Probably not many...but I, for one, do.

There are many more lessons we can learn in our suffering but one main KEY IS OUR MENTAL ATTITUDE!

If we are angry and bitter we will not learn a thing. We will only make life for those around us, miserable. If we aren't willing to do the hard work of recovery, we will remain stuck in our circumstances. If we complain or blame others for what we are going through, we will only drive people away from us.

Once again, OUR MENTAL ATTITUDE IS THE KEY TO OUR VICTORY! Even when we are trusting God for our healing, it is our attitude that will make all the difference.

Actually, our mental attitude will reveal whether or not we are TRULY trusting God.

BELIEVING IN THE WORD OF GOD

*"All Scripture is inspired by God
and profitable
for teaching,
for reprimanding,
for correction,
for training in righteousness,
so that the man of God
may be suitable
and equipped
for every good work."*

2 Timothy 3:16 & 1

At twelve years of age, I read the Bible all the way through starting in Genesis. Since then I have read the whole Bible many times. The significant thing was that, at this age, I didn't have any preconceived ideas about the Scriptures. I was able to read them with a "clear" mind, not one that had been fed by other people's opinions or with church "doctrines".

For this I am thankful!

What I am about to tell you may go against things you have been "taught in church". I hope you will think about what I say here though. Don't let "church teaching" get in the way of the truth of the Scriptures.

Reading the Bible with a "clear mind" has enabled me to "see" differently that a lot of people. I put the truth of Scripture above the "doctrine" of any church. Scripture will explain Scripture if you take the time to search it for answers. I have noticed though, so much that is being taught in Christianity is only someone's opinion. Often, one or two Scriptures are singled out to "prove" a point. This is not wise because you need the WHOLE counsel of God's Word to "put it all together" and "come to the knowledge of the truth".

The "whole counsel of God's Word" means that ALL Scripture is of equal significance. A great error being taught in Christianity is, "We don't need the Old Testament anymore. Jesus came and fulfilled the Law so it is now done away with."

THIS is a big problem with much of the teaching in Christianity today. When Christians are taught that the "Law" has been "done away with", they immediately put themselves in danger of misinterpreting Scripture.

First off the word "Law" is not a correct translation of the Hebrew word "Torah". Torah actually means "instruction" or "shooting as towards a target"! When someone teaches a lesson he or she IS "shooting towards a target", that of instilling information into the learner.

Think about this.

If we "do away" with GOD's INSTRUCTIONS what do we have left? If we do not "hit the mark" what are we doing?

MISSING THE MARK! We are, in fact, in error and disobedience.

I realize this will "fly in the face" of much of what Christians have been taught but I am all about the truth. Without the truth, we have nothing.

Now, because Torah means instruction, we should be trying to understand these instructions so we can "hit the mark". Why did God give them to us? Christians would do well to try and understand the Hebrew background to the Scriptures. Christians can learn a lot of truth about Biblical interpretation from Jewish sources.

Think about this! In the days and years immediately following the time of Y'shuah (Jesus), His early followers were almost ALL Jews! Not until the apostle Paul started reaching outside Israel with the Good News of the Messiah Y'shuah (Jesus), did a great number of Gentiles (non Jews) come to faith in Him. Before that, only the Gentiles who lived in Israel or were there to visit, were exposed to the teachings of Y'shuah (Jesus). In addition, the early Believers all met in the Synagogue on Shabbat THEN met together in the evening after the Shabbat service. See Acts 20:7-12. This talks about "meeting on the first day of the week to break bread" and how Paul "talked until midnight". In the Jewish way of reckoning a day, every day starts at sundown. This being the case, these verses are talking about meeting in the evening after the Shabbat service. This would still be our Saturday but on a Jewish calendar it is actually the beginning of the First Day of the week. Not understanding the Jewish reckoning of days has caused this confusion, thinking the Believers in Y'shuah (Jesus) actually met the day after the Shabbat.

It may seem like I am going into a lot of explanation of things that are irrelevant to healing. Not so. I am showing the continuity and relevancy of ALL Scripture. And this is going to be EXCEEDINGLY important to the understanding of this book. And to your healing.

Look again at the Scripture verses I put at the beginning of this chapter, 2 Timothy 3:16&17. You must remember, when Paul wrote this letter to Timothy, THE ONLY SCRIPTURES THEY HAD WERE WHAT CHRISTIANS KNOW AS THE OLD TESTAMENT. THERE WERE NO OTHER SCRIPTURES. This being the case, whatever is in the "New Testament" MUST AGREE WITH ALL OTHER SCRIPTURE. NONE OF IT HAS BEEN DONE AWAY WITH.

When you tie Scripture to Scripture, you will get the full and clear meaning of God's instructions to us.

15

Let me make this clear. Y'shuah (Jesus) came to set us free from death and bondage to sin. He did not set us free from the Torah or God's instructions. Salvation is by grace alone. It ALWAYS has been by grace alone. The Torah is God's instructions to us, teaching us how to relate to Him and to our fellow man AFTER we are saved by the blood Y'shuah shed on our behalf. Salvation is only the beginning. It is not the end. After being saved from the kingdom of darkness and being transferred into the Kingdom of Light, we now have the responsibility to live the rest of our lives for the one who saved us, namely YHWH (the Lord) and His Messiah, Y'shuah (Jesus). Y'shuah (Jesus) is the fullness of YHWH Himself in human form.

If you do not have your own Bible, go out and get one right away! You will need it. It will become your "life line".

In order for you to be able to tie Scripture to Scripture you will need to read and re-read the Bible many, many times. And you have to realize ALL the Scripture is relevant to today. This is why I am taking so much time in explaining these things.

The bottom line is this, THERE IS HEALING IN THE WORD OF GOD. Not just in some of the Word, but in ALL of the Word. You cannot doubt this if your healing is to come as God has intended.

Doubting the Word of God AT ALL, IN ANY WAY, will weaken your trust and in order for you to do as I did, you cannot waver in your trust of God.

LEARNING TO TRUST GOD

"One steadily thinking
upon YOU (God)
will obtain perfect peace
because in YOU (God)
he IS TRUSTING."

Isaiah 26:3

Whenever your "world" is shaken, and it will be shaken, being able to trust God will give you the strength you will need to persevere in the struggle.

This verse from Isaiah is powerful!

First, we must think STEADILY upon God. What do we think ABOUT? King David tells us in Psalms.

"Seek YHWH (the Lord)
and His strength,
seek His face continually.

Remember His wonders which He has done,
His awesome deeds..."

Psalm 105:4&5

"I shall remember
the deeds of YHWH (the Lord)!
Surely, I will remember
Your wonders of old.
I will meditate on all Your work
and think about what you have done.

Your way, O God, is set apart.
Who is like our great God?

You are the God
who works wonders!

You have made known Your strength
among the peoples.
You have, by Your power,
redeemed Your people..."

Psalm 77:11-15

First, when we read the Bible we read the testimonies of the greatness of God Almighty revealed as He dealt with the generations of Abraham, Isaac and Jacob (or Israel). From this we draw strength to trust Him in OUR own circumstances.

Next, think about your own life. Remember how God has worked in your past. It is helpful to write down the things God does for you in a book or journal. Then you can re-read them when you go through times of doubt or confusion, which we all do. When you do this you will be amazed by how many things God does for you every day!

Now I want to tell you of an important Jewish concept, the one of "Emunah".

Emunah is translated as "faith" in the English Bible. But, as is true of the Hebrew language, Emunah has a far greater meaning than the English "faith".

Emunah is what you have when you believe:

1. God is in control of ALL things. He is Sovereign and His will is always done.

2. Whatever you are going through right now, God has allowed. Nothing is beyond the grasp of God.

3. If God has allowed it, you can be certain, He has a purpose in it. And it is for your good!

Memorize these three aspects of Emunah. Remember them at all times and give God the glory no matter what circumstances you are in. We have been created to bring Him glory. This includes what you are going through right now!

"The righteousness in his 'emunah' (faith) will be."

Habakkuk 2:4

This verse is usually translated as: "The righteous shall live by faith." Now think how much more powerful is the Hebrew rendering of this verse. Hebrew is an "action" language whereas English is more "conceptual" or "abstract". There is a big difference in understanding between the two!

When we hear the word "faith" we tend to think of "belief" or "trust". All three of these words can be considered a "mind set" in English.

Not in Hebrew. "Emunah" is an action word. To have emunah is to ACT upon it! It is actually life changing and is meant to direct every aspect of a person's life.

What do I mean?

If a person believes God is in control, that whatever he or she is going through, God has allowed and not only that, but He has a PURPOSE behind it, then you can see victory after victory in your life! This is because you will not be living in confusion. You will be free to learn what God wants you to learn and you will be able to help others in a greater way as well.

The demonstration of "emunah" is found in the book of James.

"Even so
faith (emunah) without works
is dead
because it is alone."

James 2:17

In the Hebrew translation of this verse we can see that there are two sides to our "faith". One is to have the right mind set, one of trust and belief. The other is to act upon those beliefs.

This only makes sense. Our beliefs SHOULD result in actions!

If you have any doubt that God is in control, that He has

allowed your circumstances and that He has allowed them for a GOOD purpose in your life, read the book of Job. Read the Psalms. Read every book in the Bible. If your heart is open to God, you will realize the truth in having "emunah".

But, reading the Bible and praying will amount to nothing at all if you have not turned your life over to God.

Maybe you are still trying to be in control of your life. Maybe you haven't yet surrendered your life to our Almighty Creator God. If you have come to the place in your life that you want a change, that you recognize the things of the "world" are not as good as they seem to promise, if you want to be forgiven for your sins and be washed clean so you can have a new life and be with our God forever when you die, then say a prayer something like this...

Father in Heaven,
I am a sinner and I don't want to follow that path any longer.
I want to live the rest of my life for You.
I want to become the person You created me to be so my life will no longer be wasted living for myself, but for Your glory.
Please forgive me for all the bad things I have done, for the bad things I have said, for hurting others, for being selfish and self centered.
From now on I want You to be the center of my life.
I want to live my life on purpose, according to Your will.
Help me to understand Your Word as I read the Bible.
Help me to live what I read.
Thank you for taking my punishment upon Yourself as

You came to us in the person of Y'shuah (Jesus) and died in my place.

Yet, Y'shuah (Jesus) was resurrected from the dead!
I want to be resurrected from the dead too!
Please resurrect me right now into the new life You have for me!

Thank You, Father, by the power of the blood of Y'shuah (Jesus), our Messiah!
Amen

If you have just prayed this prayer, or one like it in your own words, you have now been transferred from the kingdom of darkness into the Kingdom of Light! You are now a son or daughter of the Living God!

Your life will never be the same, for now you have the power of the resurrection in you!....

WALK BY FAITH, NOT BY SIGHT

"Be always of good courage...
for we walk by faith (emunah)
and not by sight..."

2 Corinthians 5:7

"Now, faith (emunah)
is the assurance of things hoped for,
the evidence
of things not seen."

Hebrews 11:1

Does it sound "crazy" to "walk by faith and not by sight"?

What does it actually mean?

How can we do such a thing?

It takes faith or emunah. This means we cannot walk by faith if we don't have faith. So the question is, "How does one increase his or her faith?"

"Faith comes by hearing
therefore hear the Words of the Messiah."

Romans 10:17

This is an important verse. What ARE the "Words of the Messiah"?

Y'shuah (Jesus) came, not just to die in our place so we could be set free from bondage to sin and fear of death, but to reveal the Father's heart by demonstrating to us how to "walk out" the Torah.

Remember, Torah means "instruction". What upset Y'shuah (Jesus) about the Pharisees was that they had put so many "fences" around the Torah the heart of God couldn't be understood anymore. A "fence" is just that, a boundary. At first it seemed to be a good thing, a fence. God gave an instruction, so in order to be sure that His instruction was not broken, a boundary was put up to "protect" it. But then fences were put around fences and it came to be that to break a "fence" was considered breaking the Torah or instruction. THIS was what Y'shuah (Jesus) was against, not the Torah itself!

The "Words of the Messiah" mean a restoration to the heart of God's instructions or keeping the Word of God as He had originally intended it to be kept. Everything Y'shuah (Jesus) did was in line with the Torah. He was the "Living Word" and the Torah is the "Written Word". Both are light and life to those who follow them. They are, in fact, one and the same.

OK, back to increasing your faith. Read the Word of God, ALL of it. Then act upon it. As you do this, you will actually grow in your faith or emunah and in your ability to trust God more and more. Remember, if you don't ACT, you really don't believe.

It is very helpful to get a small notebook and keep it by your Bible. When you read God's Word, ask the Lord to show you what He is trying to teach you for that day. Then write it down. Write down His promises. Write down things He puts in your heart. Write down answers to prayers! This book will become valuable to you and you will actually be able to document your growth in faith.

As you grow in faith or emunah, you will learn to trust in the Word of God. This is why you need to approach the Bible as a starving man who desperately needs good nourishment to survive!

"Man cannot live by bread alone, but by EVERY WORD THAT PROCEEDS FROM THE MOUTH OF GOD!"

Deuteronomy 8:3 & Matthew 4:4

In the verse above, Y'shuah (Jesus) quoted Moses. This means EVERY WORD that proceeds from the mouth of God. None of the Bible has been "done away with" and this should prove it to anyone who would doubt.

Walking by faith, or emunah, and not by sight takes practice. It is not easy to do! We live in a world full of sights and sounds and to walk by faith means we have to "see" in the Spirit. We have to understand the heart of God and look at the world through His eyes! The ONLY way we can do this is to "wash" ourselves in His Word everyday. We need to do whatever it takes to get His Word inside of us. This will transform us!

When a person has a head injury or something similar, he or she usually struggles with memory problems. I sure did! DON'T SWEAT IT! YOU DO NOT HAVE TO MEMORIZE THE BIBLE! Just read it. Then read it some more. Don't focus on memorizing, that would be too stressful. Focus instead on ABSORBING it.

I think this is a very important point. So many people focus on what they have "lost" but this will keep you "stuck"! Focus on what you CAN do, not what you can't. Repetition, absorption, routines. These are so important because you are retraining your brain as you do these things.

STUDYING THE BIBLE WILL ACTUALLY RETRAIN AND HEAL YOUR BRAIN!

Don't get discouraged!

Remember, whatever you are going through right now, God has allowed it. And He has a purpose in it for you. Accept where you are in life and move forward. Don't let yourself stay "stuck" or go backwards by negative thinking!

This is why emunah or faith is so important. Without it you actually open yourself up to "attacks" in the mind. The enemy of our souls, the Adversary (satan in the Hebrew language means adversary), wants to defeat us. We are especially vulnerable when we let our spiritual guard down.

If you find yourself feeling down, defeated, discouraged, depressed...turn on some good God honoring music that magnifies the goodness and greatness of God Himself! Sing to YHWH (the Lord)! Let your mind be bathed in praise and thanksgiving for all you have, for all God has done for you!

Even if you find it hard to read the Bible for long right now, you can ALWAYS sing praises to God!

THERE IS HEALING IN SINGING SONGS OF PRAISE TO GOD!

Perhaps the greatest benefits we get from singing songs that magnify our Great God, are that they keep our focus on Him, they lift our Spirits and help us to keep a good attitude. They can increase our faith too!

Listening to songs that are based on Scripture is a way of internalizing the Word of God, thus increasing our faith. Singing them will drive the words into your Spirit! This is why it is SO IMPORTANT to have God honoring music. You don't want to fill your heart and mind with negative, sinful thoughts and desires.

I try to always have a song of praise in my mind, even now! I wake up with a different song every morning!

You can too!

POWER OF DISCIPLINE

"The road of life
is correction
through
self discipline."

Proverbs 6:23

This is the way the verse reads in the original Hebrew. Think about it.

The road of life...

is correction...

through...

self discipline.

Lets look at this carefully. What is "the road to life"? Life means "to be ALIVE". There are many people who live but are not "alive". If you read the Bible, you will see that there are two roads a person can take, the road leading to abundant life and the road leading to death, or a dead like existence.

Which do YOU want? We have to make the choice.

In Proverbs 6:23 we see that on the road of life there is need for correction. Correction from what? From many things, actually. Our thoughts need to be corrected. Our words and our actions. Corrected so they will line up with God's thoughts, His words and

His actions. Once we have submitted our life to Him, He is in the business of transforming us into the image of His Son, Y'shuah. Remember, Y'shuah came to show us how to live according to the heart of God. So to be conformed into His image means that those thoughts, words and actions of the flesh must go. This takes correction.

And it takes self discipline.

Here is the dictionary's definition of DISCIPLINE:

Training that develops self control.

Strict control to enforce obedience.

Orderly conduct.

Development.

Exercise.

Drilling.

Restraint.

Limitation.

Mental, physical, emotional and spiritual training.

Now tell me, does any of this sound EASY???

No.

The first step to becoming a disciplined person is that you have to WANT it. You have to be so committed to the program of discipline that you will force yourself to "tough it out" when need be.

All discipline takes MENTAL TOUGHNESS.

Let's say, right now you are not too mentally tough. How do you develop it?

First off, if this is you, don't be too concerned. Many people are not naturally mentally tough. It take practice. It takes perseverance. And, I will repeat, YOU HAVE TO WANT IT.

*"All discipline
for the moment seems
not joyful but sorrowful,
yet
to those who have been trained by it,
in the end
it will yield the peaceable fruit
of righteousness."*

Hebrews 12:11

Whatever way you look at it, discipline is not easy. BUT it is the way of LIFE, AND it yields the fruit of righteousness IN our lives.

Mental toughness comes as we make a plan and then work the plan.

Sounds simple and it is. But it is not easy!

I remember in the process of my healing when I needed to get up at 1:00am or 2:00am and go running. YES, that is what I said. I would have to get up and run at those crazy times because running was the only tool I had, then, to help balance my body. If I was "out of whack" in the middle of the night I would go run until my body got back in balance! It worked. I was determined to do whatever it took to heal my body.

Mental toughness requires determination. Once again, YOU HAVE TO WANT YOUR HEALING.

Everyone's situation is different. Ask God to help YOU to be creative to bring about your healing. Remember, God is trying to teach you many things through what you are experiencing right now.

OK, now think of the "correction" part of the verse above. What needs to be corrected in YOUR life to conform you into the image of the Messiah??

This is important.

Get out a piece of paper and draw a line down the middle of it. Put a heading on the left side: Negative. Then put a heading on the right side: Positive.

Now, pray. Ask God what are all the negative character qualities in you that He wants to change. List them line by line on the left side of your paper under: Negative.

The next part takes more prayer. Now ask God what He wants to transform those negative traits into. What positive trait does He want to develop in you as He rids you of the negative one?

For example, Anger can become Patience. Or it can become Understanding. Even Peaceful. Each person is different. The question is, what is God working out in YOUR LIFE?

This list is an important one so don't pass by this exercise.

Once you have your list done, go to your Bible and find verses that support the transformation that God is doing in you. Many of these verses will be found in Proverbs and many in Psalms. Keep searching as you read each day and write these verses down on your paper with the lists on it. MEDITATE ON THESE VERSES BECAUSE THESE ARE GOD'S WORDS TO YOU!

When you search the Scriptures like this you are, not only letting God transform your character, but you are retraining and redeveloping you brain.

OK, now when you start finding verses like this, the next step is to ACT on them. Put them into practice. This is where the self discipline comes into play. YOU HAVE TO WANT IT OR YOU WILL NOT BE ABLE TO PERSEVERE AS YOU MUST TO SEE THE CHANGES TAKE PLACE!

It is MY prayer for you that you will think seriously about what I have explained in this chapter, pray about it and then do it.

You will see miracles start to happen!

"I AM PRAYER"

"V'Ani Tefillah!"

"So, I am prayer!"

Psalm 109:4

I found this verse in the Hebrew a few months ago and was amazed by it! These words are from King David who wrote most of the Psalms. They describe the close interaction between David and his Creator, the Almighty God of the Bible.

We too should be able to say, "So, I am prayer!"

But, I believe not many people can relate to this – YET!

I love this verse because it describes MY relationship to God too. If I hadn't struggled so much in my life, I am sure this would not be so. It is in the hard times that we have a choice to either draw closer to God in an attitude of trust or to turn away from Him in an attitude of mistrust and even anger.

Today, prayer is truly the most important activity in my life – even more important that reading the Bible. I say this because even when I don't have my Bible with me, I can still pray and stay in touch with God. I say "stay" in touch not "get" in touch because our prayer life should be so constant that we are never "out of touch" with our Heavenly Father.

Many books have been written about prayer and praying. But I hope to make it simple.

"Pray without ceasing,
in all things
give thanks,
for THIS is the will of God..."

1 Thessalonians 5:17 & 18

Keeping a running conversation with God in your spirit does several things.

For one, it keeps your focus on God and not on the circumstances you may be going through or the people you may be dealing with. It helps you to release these things into His Almighty Hands and it helps to keep in constant submission to His will for you.

Next, it keeps your mind and heart clean. It is hard to meditate on anything negative or sinful if you are in conversation with God.

Is this as easy as it sounds?

Not at first, but it gets easier as you practice praying.

Here are the steps I think you will find helpful in getting into this practice:

1. Realize prayer is a discipline. You have to want it and you have to be determined to persevere in it's practice. They say it takes 6 weeks to either build or break a habit. Give yourself 6 weeks to make prayer a habit.

2. If you feel a block in your spirit or in your mind to prayer, put on some Godly music. Let the music wash your mind and spirit. Then open up your Bible...

3. Go to your Bible. Open it up to the book of Psalms. Then, starting with Psalm 1, read and pray the Scriptures back to God. Don't just pray one Psalm but several a day. Then include the book of Proverbs and pray that through too.

I will give you an example using Psalm 4:

> "Answer me when I call,
> O God of my righteousness!
> You have relieved me in my distress.
> Be gracious to me
> and hear my prayer..."

Oh Heavenly Father! I am calling out to you according to Your Word! Your Word is true therefore I put my hope in Your promises! Relieve me in my struggles. I need your strength to persevere moment by moment. Give me the grace I need at this time. Hear me, O God, for all my hope is in You!

> "But I know that YHWH (the Lord)
> has set apart the gracious man for Himself.
> YHWH (the Lord)
> HEARS when I call to Him!"

Abba! (Father in Hebrew) You say in Your Word that

You set the gracious man (woman) apart for Yourself. How awesome is that! I want to be set apart for You. Help me to be gracious to everyone as You are gracious to me. Your Word says You HEAR me when I call to You! Therefore, I am confident that You are hearing my prayer right now!

"Tremble, and do not sin,
meditate in your heart upon your bed,
and be still..."

Search me O God and know my heart! Show me where I am falling short of Your will in my life. I want to walk before You with clean hands and a clean heart. Wash me, cleanse me in the power of the blood that Y'shuah shed for me! Make me pure and whole! I am still now before You and will listen to what You tell me...

This is just an example for you in how to pray the Scriptures back to God. Make them personal. I believe these are the most powerful prayers you can pray because there is power in the Word of God.

4. When you feel comfortable with praying like this, go on to praying specifically for your transformation. Get out a piece of notebook paper you wrote your negative character qualities on and what God wants to turn them into. (If you didn't do this, go back to pages 32 & 33) As you read the Bible, start to write the Bible verses that go with these character qualities, both the negative ones and the positive ones. Now, use these lists to pray through your transformation using the Word of God. It won't be

long and you will start to become a much different person.

5. Keep a prayer journal. Write down your prayers and God's answers to them.

6. Persevere. Persevere. Persevere!

Remember, transformation is a life long process and persistent prayer is a discipline to be added to your daily life.

Set apart time in your day for your Bible reading and prayer. I like to do it in the morning while I have my coffee and simple breakfast. It can take me from 45 minutes to 3 hours or more! I have the luxury of not being in a hurry with God. Everyone's schedule is different so ask God what is the best time and way for you to get into the practice of Bible study and prayer EACH DAY.

When my children were young, I didn't have as much time as I do now. Often, I would have to include them in my Bible and prayer time. I couldn't spend as much time but I accepted what I was able to do. It works that way too.

God is very creative and He will show you what to do to make your situation work in order for you to draw closer to Him.

LEARN TO LAUGH AT YOURSELF!

"A joyful heart is good medicine!

But a broken spirit dries up the bones."

Proverbs 17:22

One of the best lessons I learned in being able to persevere in my struggles back to health, was learning to laugh at myself!

What? You may ask, how can I laugh at what I am going through? I'm struggling so hard everyday! I have lost so much! What is there to laugh at?

Before I tell the story of how I came to learn to laugh at myself, I want to tell you of something valuable I learned that anyone can apply to his or her situation when you have suffered a loss of any kind.

There are three steps to freedom in your situation:

1. Grieve your losses.

2. Assess your current strengths.

3. Let God reinvent your life.

Take time to go through this process, it is very important.

Think about all you have lost. For me, I had lost my ability to think clearly. I was not even able to put my thoughts into words anymore therefore, I was not able to communicate in a healthy, intelligible way. My thoughts were very scattered.

Now, what strengths DO you have at this time. Don't worry, they can change over time as you progress in your healing. But for now, think only of what you CAN DO at the moment, not what you cannot do.

And finally, lift it all up to God in prayer. Ask Him to use your circumstances for His glory. Ask Him to reinvent your life according to His perfect plan for you.

Write these things down and re-read them so you will be able to look at your current situation in a positive light, God's Light!

Now for my story:

It's not easy having a head injury. I went through a lot, as I am sure you have. For several years, I "fought" the injury. I tried to "force" myself to recover. But, it seemed, the more I "forced" the worse I became! I did not go to doctors for help because at the time of my accident, doctors didn't know much about head injuries.

It wasn't until after I had my first child that I was desperate for help. All I could do was cry. Even when my daughter turned a year old, I still cried all the time. My body was so weak. So I sought help.

I knew my hormones must be out of balance and didn't want to be put on medication so I looked for a Naturopath doctor to go to. There was only one in the phone book at the time so I made an appointment.

The first time I went to this doctor's office, I was as usual, in tears. He took me into his office and said, "Tell me everything you are feeling. Tell me everything you are experiencing right now." I did and as I talked, he wrote. He made a list a page long of different things he thought could be wrong with me. Then he said, "We will test each one and find out what is wrong."

No lie. I had EVERYTHING on his list wrong with me! EVERYTHING! This doctor put me on several supplements and gave me a diet for hypoglycemia. He told me to start running everyday, especially when I felt like crying.

He also took X-rays of my neck to find out what injuries I had there. He determined I needed chiropractic adjustments to my neck and back. Not only was he a Naturopath doctor but a Chiropractor so he turned out to be the right doctor for me.

One day, not long after the first visit I went to this doctor's office for a chiropractic adjustment. My neck was in so much pain! But it was because my hormones were still out of balance that I was crying. An assistant had me lay on hot packs to loosen up my muscles.

It was then that the doctor's sweet wife came by. She had not met me before so she said, "Oh, honey! Don't worry! It won't hurt that much!"

Just at that moment the doctor walked by and heard his wife. Smiling, he said, "Don't mind her! She's always like that. She's OK!"

We all laughed!

It felt soooo good to be treated like I was "normal"! The doctor had said I was "OK". For some reason, it made me feel good to think I really was OK. So from then on, that is the way I thought about myself no matter what I was going through.

From then on, I have been able to laugh at myself!

Learning to laugh has served me well and it will serve you well too! It will help OTHER people accept you where you are at and they may actually treat you better.

Even if they don't, you will have joy in your heart because the truth is that, before God, you ARE OK.

UNLOCKING & CONNECTING YOUR BRAIN

"Be transformed
by the renewing of your mind..."

Romans 12:2

Throughout my recovery, God did some very unusual things. He inspired me in certain ways. He brought things into my life I would not have discovered on my own. My healing can be attributed to Him and Him alone.

One amazing occurrence when I was about thirty five years old. An acquaintance brought me a case of music cassettes to listen to. I had been very isolated in my life so I was not familiar with what kinds of music were "out there". All of this music was written and sung by various Christian artists. This is a very important aspect to what happened next.

I started playing the music. Different groups, different songs. I played them all throughout the day. Soon though, the words "became a part of me". I could relate to them in a way I could not relate to a lot of other things. I think it is because song lyrics are often picturesque. The writers use "word pictures" to be more poetic perhaps, but it was these "word pictures" that I could relate to.

I began to be able to express myself in words, the words of these songs, because of my ability to relate to them.

For about two years, my conversations with others consisted of about 80% quotes from the songs I was listening to! I loved the songs so much I would duplicate them and give them away to others so they could be blessed as I was!

The amazing thing is that these songs actually helped me connect my thoughts and feelings with my words. Something I had not been able to do up until then.

Here are some words from a song I still remember by Janny:

"Broken wings take time to mend,
before they learn to fly again…

On the breath of God they'll soar,
they'll be stronger that before…

On the breath of God I'll soar,
I'll be stronger than before!"

I think I had discovered a key to mental healing! Music. The right kind of music.

Even to this day, music is extremely important to me. It speaks to my spirit, to my soul, to my emotions, to my mind. Music is a source of amazing power in a person's life. This is why it is SO VERY IMPORTANT TO BE LISTENING TO GOD HONORING MUSIC!

I encourage you to listen to "Messianic" Christian music too! It tends to lift up the greatness of our Holy God in a powerful way that is a bit different than traditional Christian music. For example, try Paul Wilbur's or Joshua Aaron's music. I have many favorites but this would be a good place to start.

You want to fill your mind, heart, spirit and being with the TRUTH OF TH WORD OF GOD. Think of this when you listen to or buy music. Much Christian and all Messianic music is based on Scripture.

I like a lot of Jewish religious music too! Actually, there is something very healing about the Hebrew language. Scripture sung in Hebrew is powerful!

Find God honoring music YOU can relate to. Let God's Word wash over you in song! It will cleanse you and bring healing. It will help reconnect the mind and the heart. It will give you words to use in expressing yourself even if you don't have words right now.

If you really are struggling to reconnect your thoughts and feelings with your words, keep a small notebook with you. Write in it words that you hear from others but especially in the music you listen to, that express what you want to tell others. It's OK to quote music! I did for a long while. I still do, actually, if I hear words that are helpful for me today!

Remember, healing is a process. And processes take time.

The key is to keep moving FORWARD!

If you feel "stuck" or like you are going backwards, get someone to help you work through the difficultly. BUT, YOU MUST NOT BECOME DEPENDENT UPON OTHERS. In the end, this will only cripple you. Of course you may HAVE to be dependent for a while, maybe even a long while. But you should always make it your goal to become more and more INDEPENDENT, no actually it is, GOD DEPENDENT!

The more you are dependent upon God, the less you will have to be dependent upon others and the quicker you will progress in your healing!

PUTTING IT ALL TOGETHER

"Be renewed in the spirit of your mind,
and put on your new self,
which in the likeness of God
has been created
in righteousness and being set apart
in the truth."

Ephesians 4:23 & 24

I have introduced many ideas in this book that may be new to you. You may wonder how to put these ideas into action in YOUR life so you can progress on the road to healing, God's way.

First, I will tell you a little more of my own story so you can see how healing came to me.

Back in 1970 doctors did not know much about treating head injuries. I was "sewn up" and sent home to recover. My head was wrapped so the swelling wouldn't open the wound but it had to go somewhere. My eyes turned black and blue and swelled shut. What a sight I was!

As I lay in bed, I knew some changes had taken place inside my head. I was sensitive to light and noise in ways I had not been before. I couldn't follow conversations. I saw my brothers and sisters doing things but it would take me time to realize exactly WHAT they were doing. My brain worked very slowly.

I think I was in bed about two weeks before I was able to be up much. Severe injuries require a lot of time to recuperate. Rest and sleep are a part of the healing.

When I began to function a bit more, I knew things were not the same. I didn't understand it but I am not one to stay "stuck". Because of the prayers I had prayed, I realized that God had allowed this accident for a reason. I wanted to learn what I could from it. So I prayed all the time, asking God for His wisdom.

I remember thinking, "OK, I am limited, but what CAN I do?"

Then I did what I could.

I swept the kitchen floor. I did the dishes. I read recipes and cooked meals. I read my Bible and prayed.

School was almost impossible for me to complete but with the help of my teachers, I did graduate from high school. I don't remember much of that time in my life. I just know it was hard. The other students didn't know what was wrong with me. I was just very quiet. I had to focus on what GOD was doing, not what other people thought. So, I did what I could.

I ended up working on a horse race track after high school because, in my condition, I couldn't go on to college. But, as it turned out, that was the perfect place for me to be! I learned later on from a doctor, that they had discovered HARD PHYSICAL LABOR is the best way to accelerate healing for head injuries. How about that? God directed me to just the place I needed to be. Cleaning horse stalls, brushing horses and sweeping shed rows is a lot of hard physical work. Especially when you have ten to twelve horse to take care of! I was also able to rest there whenever I needed to. Actually, I felt very good working like that!

When I ended up going to the Naturopath doctor several years later, I discovered the healing power in running and in good nutrition.

Even if you can't run, go for walks. Move your body as much as possible! Keep the blood flowing! When blood is pumped into the brain, healing accelerates.

Good nutrition also helps the healing process. The hypoglycemic diet I was on is actually a healthy diet for anyone. Slowly, slowly I started to get stronger and stronger.

These are all very important aspects of healing. Rest, Hard Exercise, Good Nutrition and Positive Attitude. But, without focused Bible reading and continual prayer, I do not think I would have been able to persevere in all the other things. It is especially important to keep a positive attitude. Reading Scripture and listening to God honoring music are what has kept me moving forward and not staying "stuck". Prayer, or constant communication with God is my lifeline to Hope.

Without HOPE you have no vision for your future. Without HOPE you cannot go on, persevering through the "hard stuff" of life. How much more, when you are in the process of recovering from a head injury!

Here is Hebrews 11:1 once again:

"Now, faith (emunah)
is the assurance of things HOPED for,
the evidence
of things not seen."

Hebrews 11:1

Faith or emunah and hope are connected. Read this verse again. FAITH is the ASSURANCE of things HOPED for...even before the evidence is seen.

Practice EMUNAH or faith. What good is trusting God if you do not have the FAITH to believe in the TRUTH of His Word? I believe, THIS is the biggest key to my healing and to yours!

I want to reinforce some things I wrote about in previous

chapters. Study them, pray about them and ask God how to apply them to YOUR life, to YOUR situation.

The prayers I prayed when I was twelve:

1. I said, "God, if Your Word is true I want You to prove it true in my life."

2. I had read how the sins of the parents are passed on to the third and fourth generation so I prayed, "God, no matter what it takes, I ask that you break all the sins of my forefathers in me."

3. I realized we all have only one life to live so I asked, "God, I want my life to count. I don't want to waste it. Please use me for Your glory. I don't care what I have to go through. I just want my life to count for all eternity and for it to bring You glory."

Emunah (faith) means:

1. God is in control of ALL things. He is Sovereign and His will is always done.

2. Whatever you are going through right now, God has allowed. Nothing is beyond the grasp of God.

3. If God has allowed it, you can be certain, He has a purpose in it. And it is for your good!

The dictionary's definition of DISCIPLINE:

Training that develops self control.

Strict control to enforce obedience.

Orderly conduct.

Development.

Exercise.

Drilling.

Restraint.

Limitation.

Mental, physical, emotional and spiritual training.

Learning to LIVE IN THE PRESENCE OF GOD:

1. Realize prayer is a discipline. You have to want it and you have to be determined to persevere in it's practice. They say it takes 6 weeks to either build or break a habit. Give yourself 6 weeks to make prayer a habit.

2. If you feel a block in your spirit or in your mind to prayer, put on some Godly music. Let the music wash your mind and spirit. Then open up your Bible...

3. Go to your Bible. Open it up to the book of Psalms. Then, starting with Psalm 1, read and pray the Scriptures back to God. Don't just pray one Psalm but several a day. Then include the book of Proverbs and pray that through too.

I will give you an example using Psalm 4:

"Answer me when I call,
O God of my righteousness!

You have relieved me in my distress.
Be gracious to me
and hear my prayer..."

Oh Heavenly Father! I am calling out to you according to Your Word! Your Word is true therefore I put my hope in Your promises! Relieve me in my struggles. I need you strength to persevere moment by moment. Give me the grace I need at this time. Hear me, O God, for all my hope is in You!

"But I know that YHWH (the Lord)
has set apart the gracious man for Himself.
YHWH (the Lord)
HEARS when I call to Him!"

Abba! (Father in Hebrew) You say in Your Word that You set the gracious man (woman) apart for Yourself. How awesome is that! I want to be set apart for You. Help me to be gracious to everyone as You are gracious to me. Your Word say You HEAR me when I call to You! Therefore, I am confident that You are hearing my prayer right now!

"Tremble, and do not sin,
meditate in your heart upon your bed,
and be still..."

Search my O God and know my heart! Show me where I am falling short of Your will in my life. I want to walk before You with clean hands and a clean heart. Wash me, cleanse me in the power of the blood that Y'shuah shed for me! Make me pure and whole! I am still now before You and will listen to what You tell me...

This is just an example for you in how to pray the Scriptures back to God. I believe these are the most powerful prayers you can pray because there is power in the Word of God.

4. When you feel comfortable with praying like this, go on to praying specifically for your transformation. Get out a piece of notebook paper you wrote your negative character qualities on and what God wants to turn them into. (If you didn't do this, go back to pages 31 & 32) As you read the Bible, start to write the Bible verses that go with these character qualities, both the negative ones and the positive ones. Now, use these lists to pray through your transformation using the Word of God. It won't be long and you will become a much different person.

5. Keep a prayer journal. Write down your prayers and God's answers to them.

6. Persevere. Persevere. Persevere!

Three steps to freedom in any situation:

1. Grieve your losses.

2. Assess your current strengths.

3. Let God reinvent your life.

Recovery is not an easy process. It takes determination and perseverance and most of all faith. I believe you will receive your healing as you pursue God's purposes in your life.

Keep a notebook on your recovery.

Here is something to remember from 2 Corinthians:

"Blessed be the God and Father
of our Lord, Y'shuah (Jesus) the Messiah,
the Father of mercies

and God of all comfort,
who comforts us
in all our afflictions
so that
we will be able to comfort
those who are in any affliction
with the comfort
with which we ourselves
are comforted
by God."

2 Corinthians 1:3&4

We go through afflictions so God can walk with us through them. THEN we are to walk with others in their afflictions, comforting them as God Himself comforted us.

This means, that whatever God has allowed you to go through, He has a purpose in it and He will redeem it when you submit yourself to His perfect plan for your life.

BE A BLESSING, REACH OUT TO OTHERS

"YHWH (the Lord)
restored the fortunes of Job
when he prayed
for his friends..."

Job 42:10

I cannot finish this book without mentioning the importance of reaching out to others, even as you are in the process of recovery yourself.

Look at this verse from the book of Job.

Job was restored, his health and all that he had lost, when he got his eyes off of himself and prayed for his friends.

We are to do the same.

Think of someone in a worse situation than yourself. Pray for that person.

Think of how YOU can bless someone today, everyday! Even if it is only a smile and a kind word. You can do something for someone else.

This may even develop into a ministry for you. It did for me, several times!

HEALING WILL COME
WHEN YOU ASK GOD HOW HE CAN USE YOU
IN THE LIVES OF OTHERS

TO BRING BLESSING TO THEM!

I cannot emphasize this enough. Read the whole book of Job. Read it in one sitting if you can and you will surely be blessed.

Pray the Psalms into other people's lives and see miracles happen! For you and for them!

END NOTE

*"And we know
that God
causes ALL things
to work together for good
to those who love God,
to those who are called
according to His purposes.*

*For those whom He foreknew,
He also predestined
to be conformed
into the image of His Son."*

Romans 8:28 & 29

I want to say something to encourage each and everyone who reads this book. God is in control. He has all the power of the universe at His command. He CAN heal you in a moment's time but if He has chosen you to go through a process in order for you to become the man or woman He created you to be, then submit to His process and God will use you in amazing ways.

Each one of us was created for specific purposes. But we have choices to make. Do we have the courage to let go of living a selfish, self centered life and turn it over to God so He can use us in the greatest possible way? Are we willing to become a "Living Sacrifice"? Can we "Let go and Let God" work?

I believe with all my heart and being that if you follow the process God led me through, you will see miracles happen in your own life! And you will become a blessing to those around you. What more can you ask for?

I want to leave you with a sort of "Check List" to remind you in a simple, easy way what steps to take to receive your healing from God. Sometimes God brings instant healing! But sometimes healing is a God ordained process.

Pray for instant but submit to the process!

1. Believe in the truth of the Word of God.

2. Commit your life to the One who Created you and who holds the world in His hands by surrendering your life to Him and to Messiah Y'shuah (Jesus), God coming in the flesh, who died to save your soul and set you free.

3. Buy yourself a good Bible and read in it everyday. Read all of it but be sure to read in the Psalms and Proverbs each day as well.

4. Pray God's Word back to Him. Spend time listening to what He has to say to you.

5. Make a list of your negative character qualities and the positive ones God wants to transform them into.
Collect Scriptures to back you up.
Then pray these Scriptures back to God.

6. Work on your emunah or faith. Trust God in the darkness of your circumstances. Remember, even the night is day to Him!

7. Walk by faith and not by sight. Don't be deceived by what you see. Look ahead to what God is doing.

8. Practice being Disciplined in your daily life.

9. Learn to laugh at yourself and your circumstances.

10. Reach out to others. Focus on being a blessing to everyone God brings into your life!

Remember what I said in a previous chapter, if you want to get what God has for you in life, in every situation, you have to ask the right questions. Not, "Why me?" But, "What are You trying to teach me through this?" This will make all the difference in the outcome of your times of struggle.

"If YHWH (the Lord) had not been my help,
my soul would soon have dwelt
in silence...

When my anxious thoughts
multiply within me,
Your comfort
delights my soul."

Psalm 94:17&19

www.ingramcontent.com/pod-product-compliance
Lightning Source LLC
Chambersburg PA
CBHW071244280526
45788CB00004B/1583